THE **SCIENCE**
OF **VITAMIN D**

EVERYTHING YOU NEED TO KNOW ABOUT VITAMIN D

LA FONCEUR

Eb
emerald books

Eb
emerald books

Copyright © 2024 La Fonceur

ISBN: 978-93-340-2238-4

All rights reserved. No part of this publication may be reproduced, stored in a retrieval system or transmitted in any form or by any means, electronic, mechanical, photocopying, recording or otherwise, without prior permission of author.

Cover art illustrated by Famenxt

This book has been published with all efforts taken to make the material error-free. The information on this book is not intended or implied to be a substitute for diagnosis, prognosis, treatment, prescription, and/or dietary advice from a licensed health professional. Author and publisher don't assume and hereby disclaim any liability to any party for any loss, damage, or disruption caused by errors or omissions, whether such errors or omissions result from negligence, accident, or any other cause.

While every effort has been made to avoid any mistake or omission, this publication is being sold on the condition and understanding that neither the author nor the publishers or printers would be liable in any manner to any person by reason of any mistake or omission in this publication or for any action taken or omitted to be taken or advice rendered or accepted on the basis of this work.

CONTENTS

Introduction 5

Chapter 1: Basics of Vitamin D 7

Chapter 2: Food Fortification 15

Chapter 3: Everything You Need to Know About Vitamin D 20

Chapter 4: Importance of Vitamin D 35

Chapter 5: 10 Natural Sources to Get Vitamin D ... 47

Chapter 6: Potentially Dangerous Vitamin D Combinations You Should Avoid 55

Chapter 7: Vitamin D Combinations for Synergistic Health Benefits 58

Chapter 8: Diet Plan 64

Chapter 9: Recipes 65

Pan Fried Cheesy Mushrooms *66*

Stuffed Bell Pepper *68*

Contents

Kiwi Smoothie *70*

Read Books of the Eat So What! Series 71

References 72

About the Author 81

Read More from La Fonceur 82

Connect with La Fonceur 82

Color Your Vitamin D 83

INTRODUCTION

Although you may have some knowledge about vitamin D, your awareness is probably limited to what you've heard from health advocates or dietary supplement manufacturing companies. You may come across countless articles promoting the benefits of vitamins, and they often conclude with recommendations for specific supplements.

Dietary supplements have become easily accessible and convenient, saving time and effort. Many rely on supplements due to a busy lifestyle and limited knowledge about what their body needs for optimal health. This dependence may result in an unwillingness to obtain essential nutrients from natural sources.

When questioned about the benefits of vitamin D, the usual response from most individuals would be vitamin D is good for bone health. However, vitamin D does much more than that. Taking vitamin D from natural sources can provide various other health benefits that may surprise you. In fact, this vitamin has been known to affect your health in numerous ways, some of which are yet to be fully discovered. This is why relying on vitamin supplements may not provide the same results that can be effortlessly obtained through natural sources. If you're not focusing on getting vitamin D through natural sources, you're missing out on a lot of potential health benefits.

Get all your answers about vitamin D with the ***The Science of Vitamin D*** book. Learn about its crucial role in maintaining good health and the latest scientific findings and how this can affect your vitamin decisions. Learn in detail about fortified foods and whether or not you should take them. Clear up common vitamin-related dilemmas, such as how to tell if you're deficient in vitamin D and when to get tested.

Learn about the advantages of combining vitamin D with other vitamins and minerals for optimal health benefits, as well as the potential consequences of taking vitamin D with certain foods or medications. This guide covers both beneficial and harmful combinations of vitamin D, as well as the advantages and drawbacks of fortified foods and vitamin supplements.

Furthermore, learn about natural sources that are high in vitamin D. By consuming these foods and lifestyle changes, you can avoid vitamin D deficiencies and maintain good overall health, reducing the likelihood of infections and chronic illnesses such as cancer, diabetes, high blood pressure, and cognitive decline. Plus, explore some nutritious and easy-to-cook vegetarian recipes that can be included in your diet to maximize the health benefits of vitamin D.

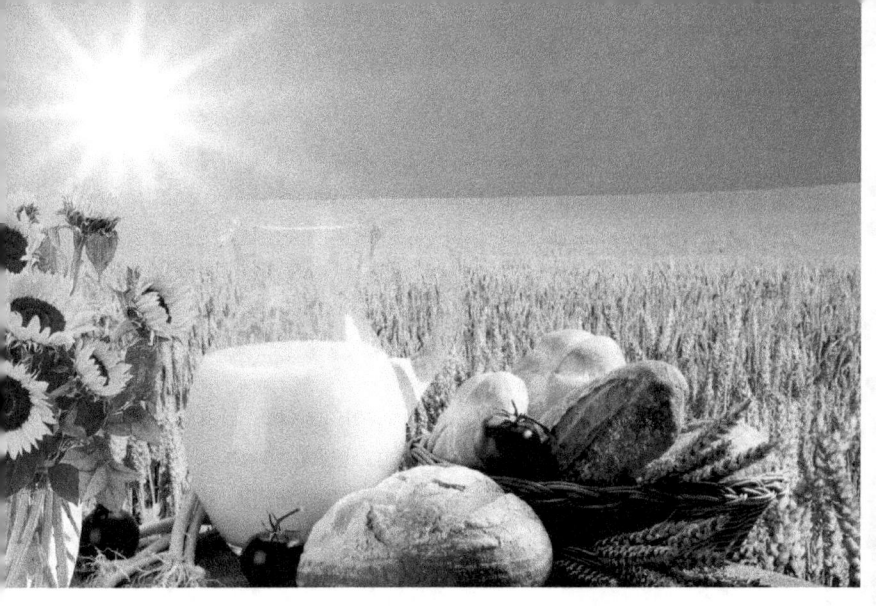

CHAPTER 1

BASICS OF VITAMIN D

Vitamins are organic compounds required by the body in small quantities to perform various normal functions Vitamins can be essential or non-essential. Essential nutrients are crucial for the normal function of the body, and the body cannot produce them, so they must be obtained through food.

Vitamins differ from macronutrients such as carbohydrates, proteins, and fats because they do not provide energy and are required in smaller quantities. They are called micronutrients because they are needed in small amounts, but this does not make them any less important than macronutrients.

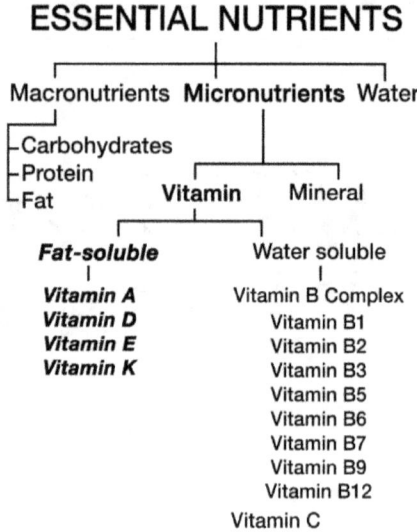

While vitamins are now a topic of general discussion, it may surprise you that they were discovered not so long ago. In fact, all known vitamins were identified during the period between 1912 and 1948.

CLASSIFICATION OF ESSENTIAL VITAMINS

There are 13 essential vitamins that are classified as water-soluble vitamins and fat-soluble vitamins.

Water-Soluble Vitamins

Water-soluble Vitamins are Vitamin B1, B2, B3, B4, B5, B6, B7, B12 and Vitamin C. These vitamins are called water-soluble as they dissolve in water. There are nine of them, including Vitamin B1 to B12 and Vitamin C. Since they dissolve in water, they are easily absorbed, and any excess is excreted in urine quickly without being stored in the body. This is why it is essential to consume water-soluble vitamins regularly to maintain adequate levels.

Fat-Soluble Vitamins

Fat-soluble vitamins are Vitamin A, Vitamin D, Vitamin E and Vitamin K. Fat-soluble vitamins are not soluble in water but instead, dissolve in fats. There are five vitamins that are classified as fat-soluble vitamins - vitamins A, D, E, and K, and these are absorbed by the body in a similar way to dietary fats. When you consume fat-soluble vitamins with healthy fats, their absorption in the intestine increases. Unlike water-soluble vitamins, fat-soluble vitamins are stored in the body and can be used whenever the body requires them. The body stores fat-soluble vitamins in the liver, muscles, and fatty tissue (adipocytes). This means that a continuous supply of fat-soluble vitamins is not necessary, as they are not excreted from the body as quickly as water-soluble vitamins. However, consuming adequate amounts is important to reach the daily recommended intake.

Too much of vitamin D can lead to toxicity (Hypervitaminosis). Toxicity usually occurs when taking supplements, not from food. A balanced diet typically provides sufficient amounts of fat-soluble vitamins. The following chapters will discuss vitamins D in detail.

Which vitamin deficiency is most common?

Surprisingly, vitamin D deficiency is currently one of the most common vitamin deficiencies worldwide and has become a global concern with serious health consequences. This deficiency is a reflection of our lifestyle and indiscipline. Although out-of-control risk factors such as aging and malabsorption syndromes cannot be controlled, other undisciplined lifestyle choices such as sedentariness, lack of sunlight, and obesity as well as poor food choices can be easily acted upon and successfully prevent Vitamin D deficiency.

Types of Vitamin Deficiency

There are two types of vitamin deficiency:

Primary deficiency
Secondary deficiency

Primary deficiency

Primary deficiency can happen when you do not eat enough foods that are high in vitamins.

Reasons:

- Poor diet.
- Unavailability of a particular vitamin-rich food in that region.

Secondary deficiency

A secondary deficiency can happen when the body cannot properly absorb or use vitamins.

Reasons:

- Poor lifestyle choices such as smoking and drinking alcohol.
- Use of medications that interfere with the absorption of vitamins.
- An underlying disorder that limits the absorption of vitamins.

What is Oxidative Stress and Antioxidants?

Oxidative processes are normal in the body and are important to provide energy for many cellular functions. Oxygen is used by cells to generate energy, with free radicals being produced as a by-product. In small amounts, free radicals are beneficial as they can kill pathogens and regulate cell growth and death. However, excessive free radicals can cause chronic diseases. The body produces free radicals during normal cell metabolism, but external sources like radiation, pollution, cigarette smoke, and medication can also expose you to these harmful free radicals. Drinking alcohol and consuming excess sugar, and fat may also contribute to free radical production.

Free radicals are unpaired electrons that like to be paired. Antioxidants are produced by the body to balance free radicals and stop them from causing damage. Oxidative stress occurs when there is an imbalance between free radicals and antioxidants, and the accumulation of free radicals in the body cannot be gradually eliminated. This process causes unpaired free radicals to pair with electrons in fat tissue, proteins, and DNA, and this can damage cells and tissues, increasing the risk of developing chronic and degenerative diseases like cancer, rheumatoid arthritis, cataracts, diabetes, aging, as well as cardiovascular and neurodegenerative diseases.

Some foods have antioxidant properties and can delay or inhibit cellular damage by their free radical scavenging ability. These antioxidant foods are capable of breaking the free radical chain reaction by donating an electron to a free radical without destabilizing themselves. The three vitamins that act as antioxidants are pro-vitamin A (carotenoids), vitamin E, and vitamin C. Since these micronutrients cannot be produced by the body, they must be obtained through the diet.

Recent research indicates that Vitamin D exhibits antioxidant properties and have the potential to manage and prevent diseases. However, further studies are necessary to determine their exact role as antioxidants.

What is Inflammation and Anti-inflammatory?

Let's first understand what is inflammation:

Is inflammation good or bad?

Both. The process of inflammation is a natural defense mechanism of the body. It is the process by which the immune system identifies and eliminates harmful and foreign bodies, and begins the healing process. there are two types of inflammation, acute inflammation, which lasts for a few days, is helpful in cases where the body experiences injury or harm. For instance, if you have a cut on your finger, your body sends inflammatory cells to the injury site to start the healing process.

Chronic inflammation is a type of inflammation that occurs over a longer period of time and can last for several months or even years. Even when there is no external threat, your body continues to send inflammatory cells, which can create an ongoing and unnecessary inflammatory condition. This can eventually harm healthy tissues in the long run. Chronic inflammation is the primary cause of many chronic diseases, including rheumatoid arthritis, chronic obstructive pulmonary disease (COPD), diabetes, and cancer.

Chronic inflammation can be caused by several factors, including environmental pollutants, auto-immune diseases, infection, and untreated acute inflammation. Lifestyle factors, such as stress, obesity, alcohol consumption, and smoking, can also contribute to inflammation in the body. It is crucial to treat inflammation promptly, as not doing so can result in life-threatening consequences. Vitamin D is anti-inflammatory and has a specific pathway to reduce inflammation in the body, which will be discussed in detail in chapter 4.

Is vitamin D a non-essential vitamin?

Non-essential vitamins are the vitamins that the body can make. Most vitamins are essential and cannot be produced by the body, except for vitamins D, K, and B7.

The skin produces Vitamin D when exposed to certain UVB rays from direct sunlight. Although technically non-essential, vitamin D is still considered essential nutrients because it plays a crucial role in the normal growth and development of the body.

CHAPTER 2

FOOD FORTIFICATION

What is food fortification?

Food fortification and food enrichment sound similar but are different. Both involve adding essential nutrients such as vitamins and minerals to food and share the common goal of preventing nutritional deficiencies and promoting public health while minimizing potential health risks. However, food enrichment adds back essential nutrients lost during processing, while fortification adds additional essential nutrients that may not be present or only present in small amounts prior to processing.

Types of Fortifications:

Mandatory Fortification is when governments legally oblige food manufacturers to add certain vitamins or minerals, or both, to specified foods. Common examples of mandatory fortifications are the addition of iodine in salt, vitamins—riboflavin, thiamin, and niacin to flour, and vitamins A and D to milk.

Voluntary Fortification allows food producers to add vitamins or minerals, or both, to foods, as long as they comply with the regulatory guidelines of the country. Common examples of voluntary fortifications are breakfast cereal and soy milk.

Are these added micronutrients natural?

These added micronutrients are either derived from plants or animals, or they are synthetic, artificial chemicals created in a laboratory. Food manufacturers add these chemicals to their products during production which contain vitamins and minerals.

How are fortified foods different from dietary supplements?

A dietary supplement is any product that supplements the diet. It can come in the form of a concentrate, extract, metabolite, or combination and may contain vitamins, minerals, amino acids, herbs, or other botanical substances. However, unlike drugs, the effectiveness and safety of supplements are not tested.

Fortified foods and dietary supplements both strive to enhance the nutrition of individuals. Fortified foods contain a mild vitamins and minerals, while supplements utilize concentrated nutrients. Fortification aims to boost the nutritional value of individuals, while supplementation works to rectify any nutritional deficiencies in a person.

Why is food fortification necessary when all the essential nutrients are available through natural food sources?

Fortification is necessary due to poor diet, insufficient essential nutrients in the diet, and the unavailability of certain foods in some areas of the world. Iodized salt is the most crucial and effective fortification for preventing goiter.

Another reason for fortification is the extensive processed food available in the market. This processing is done to enhance the taste and increase the shelf life of the product, but it results in the loss of vital vitamins and minerals. The fortification of food ensures that these lost nutrients are added back to the food.

In order to avoid relying on fortified foods or supplements, it is important to have knowledge of which foods contain specific nutrients, the recommended daily intake of each nutrient, and the ideal combination of foods to achieve optimal nutrition.

Who benefits most from food fortification?

Elderly people and pregnant women have higher nutritional needs. Therefore, fortified foods can meet their increased nutritional demands. Fortified foods are also beneficial for people who have certain food allergies or who follow restricted diets.

How do I know if a food is fortified or not?

Always check the nutrition label of your packaged foods. This label will provide details about any added nutrients. If the label specifies that certain essential nutrients have been added, then that food has been fortified.

Is it safe to consume fortified food?

It is generally safe to consume fortified foods, but it is important to note that they should not be relied upon as the sole source of nutrients. Fortification is meant to provide micronutrients that are typically found in a well-balanced diet. While fortified foods may contain higher levels of certain micronutrients, they cannot replace a healthy diet that includes sufficient carbohydrates, protein, essential fats, and other nutrients for optimal health.

Consuming a variety of fortified foods throughout the day can even lead to nutrient overdoses, particularly in children. Many fortified foods available in the market contain levels of vitamins that are not appropriate for children, which can be potentially dangerous.

Is fortified food good or bad?

The food industry often markets highly processed and sugary items as " fortified with essential nutrients," leading people to believe they are making healthy choices. However, these foods are often high in salt, trans fats, saturated fats, and sugar. Simply fortifying a food item does not necessarily make it healthy or beneficial for your health. While micronutrient intake is crucial, healthy food should not just offer essential nutrients but also be low in sugar, salt, trans fats, and saturated fats.

While fortified foods can certainly be included in a healthy diet, they are not sufficient by themselves. You cannot rely on fortified foods to get all the nutrients you need. Your body still needs a complete diet that is rich in fruits and vegetables of different colors along with whole grains and legumes to keep you strong and healthy.

CHAPTER 3

EVERYTHING YOU NEED TO KNOW ABOUT VITAMIN D

Vitamin D is a fat-soluble essential vitamin, which is also known as calciferol. It is present in certain natural foods and can also be synthesized by the body when your skin is exposed to a certain range of ultraviolet rays from sunlight, which trigger vitamin D synthesis.

Vitamin D cannot technically be considered an "essential" vitamin as it can be synthesized by the body. Non-essential doesn't mean it is not important, it simply means that your body can produce it, and you do not need to rely solely on food sources.

Read more about essential and non-essential nutrients in Eat So What! The Power of Vegetarianism.

Forms of Vitamin D

Vitamin D3 (cholecalciferol) and vitamin D2 (ergocalciferol) are the two most important forms of vitamin D for your health.

Vitamin D3 or Cholecalciferol (Animal-based) – It is naturally synthesized by animals, including humans. When your skin is exposed to ultraviolet rays from sunlight, it synthesizes cholecalciferol in the lower layers of the epidermis (skin) through a chemical reaction. Vitamin D3 is slightly more active than Vitamin D2.

Vitamin D2 or Ergocalciferol (Plant-based) – It can be found in food and is also used as a dietary supplement. Just like humans, some foods, such as mushrooms, make Vitamin D when exposed to ultraviolet light. The difference is our skin makes Vitamin D3, while mushrooms produce Vitamin D2 when exposed to ultraviolet rays of sunlight.

Vitamin D obtained from sun exposure and foods, i.e., both Vitamin D2 and D3 are biologically inactive and must get activated in the body. The first activation occurs in the liver, which converts vitamin D to 25-hydroxyvitamin D or 25(OH)D or, simply known as calcifediol. The second activation occurs primarily in the kidney and forms the physiologically active 1,25-dihydroxyvitamin D or 1,25(OH)2D or, simply known as calcitriol.

Which is more important for me, Vitamin D2 or D3?

Vitamin D3 and D2 both are important to health. So, you need both forms equally. However, it has been found that Vitamin D3 (cholecalciferol) is slightly more effective than Vitamin D2 (ergocalciferol) in increasing blood concentrations of the vitamin, and with the same daily doses of vitamin D2 and D3, calcifediol blood levels increased by vitamin D2 declined faster than the vitamin D3. So, it is basically Vitamin D3 that maintains the required levels of Vitamin D in your body. That makes getting sunlight even more crucial than obtaining Vitamin D from other sources. However, this does not diminish the importance of Vitamin D2. Both forms are equally important, but obtaining Vitamin D through sunlight can maintain your vitamin D levels for a longer period, and you get the maximum health benefits of vitamin D.

How much vitamin D do I need in a day?

The average daily recommended intake of vitamin D that is sufficient to meet the nutrient needs of nearly all (97%–98%) healthy individuals is:

Age 0-12 months – 400 IU (10 mcg) [Adequate Intake (AI)]

Age 1 - 70 years – 600 IU (15 mcg)

Age 70+ years – 800 IU (20 mcg)

*1 mcg is equal to 40 IU

How common is Vitamin D deficiency?

It would seem that Vitamin D is probably the easiest nutrient to get because it doesn't even need to depend on food, and you can easily get it from the sunlight, but in reality, about 50% of the world's population is vitamin D deficient. One of the most prevalent reasons for this is that many individuals do not receive adequate sunlight. This could be due to spending more time indoors and applying sunscreen before going outdoors.

What are the reasons that lead to a deficiency in Vitamin D?

- You are not getting enough sunlight exposure.
- Your diet might be lacking in vitamin D.

- You might have a malabsorption problem, which makes your body unable to absorb enough vitamin D from food.

- You live in a colder area.

- Your liver or kidneys are unable to convert vitamin D to its active form as all vitamin D forms are inactive in general and get activated in the liver and kidney.

- You have had weight loss surgery.

- You might be taking other medications that are interfering with how your body converts or absorbs vitamin D.

- You have certain medical conditions, such as liver disease or kidney disease.

What are the risk factors associated with vitamin D deficiency?

Fat Malabsorption: Fat malabsorption is a condition where your body is unable to absorb certain nutrients from your diet, even if you eat nutrient-dense foods. This can be caused by various factors such as lactose intolerance, prolonged use of antibiotics, damage to the intestine due to infection, inflammation or surgery, certain medical conditions, and radiation therapy. Vitamin D is a fat-soluble nutrient, which means that its absorption depends on the intestine's ability to absorb dietary fat. If you have difficulty absorbing dietary fat, your vitamin D levels might be low, and you may need to take vitamin D supplements.

Obesity: Studies have found that people who have a body mass index (BMI) of 30 or higher tend to have lower vitamin D levels than lean people. While obesity does not hinder your skin's ability to produce vitamin D, having more subcutaneous fat can absorb more of the vitamin, making it less available in the body. Therefore, People who are obese need to consume more vitamin D in order to achieve similar levels to those with a normal weight.

Gastric Bypass Surgery: Individuals who are obese and have had a gastric bypass surgery may become vitamin D deficient. It is because, during this procedure, a portion of the upper small intestine responsible for absorbing vitamin D is bypassed. As a result, vitamin D that is released from fat stores into the bloodstream may not elevate the levels of 25(OH)D (the active form of vitamin D) to a sufficient level over time.

Kidney or Liver Disease: Kidney or liver disease can affect your body's ability to convert inactive vitamin D into active forms for use.

Certain Medical Conditions: Some medical conditions like certain liver diseases, celiac disease, Crohn's disease, cystic fibrosis, and ulcerative colitis can lead to fat malabsorption. This affects the gut's ability to absorb vitamin D from food. Individuals with these conditions have a higher risk of vitamin D deficiency. Because of these conditions, they may also avoid certain foods like dairy products or consume them in small amounts, which can contribute to vitamin D deficiency.

Certain Medications: Using stimulant laxatives for an extended period can decrease the body's ability to absorb vitamin D from food, and taking high doses can even lead to osteomalacia.

Individuals who take oral antidiabetic medication typically have lower levels of vitamin D compared to those with diabetes who do not take these drugs.

Other medications that affect vitamin D status are steroids, weight-loss drugs, anti-seizure drugs, antivirals, antidepressants, anti-hypertensive drugs, vitamin K antagonists, and bile acid sequestrants.

What health problems can occur from Vitamin D deficiency?

Low blood levels of vitamin D are associated with the following conditions:

Hypocalcemia

Low levels of calcium in your blood can result in a condition known as hypocalcemia. Having sufficient levels of calcium is essential for maintaining strong and healthy bones, as well as a healthy functioning heart. When the body lacks vitamin D, your body cannot absorb enough calcium to meet its requirements. Therefore, a deficiency in vitamin D can cause low calcium levels in the blood, which can result in weakened bones and impact cardiovascular health.

Hypophosphatemia

If your body has low levels of phosphate, you may have a short-term or chronic condition called hypophosphatemia. Phosphate is vital for building and repairing bones and teeth, enabling muscle contraction, and ensuring nerve function. While vitamin D status doesn't directly impact phosphate levels, it can indirectly affect them. A lack of vitamin D in the body reduces calcium absorption, causing hypocalcemia. This, in turn, stimulates the secretion of parathyroid hormone (PTH) to fix the hypocalcemia by acting on bone and kidney. However, it also increases urinary phosphate excretion, leading to hypophosphatemia and osteomalacia.

Rickets

Rickets is a medical condition that primarily affects children and results in softening and weakening of the bones. This is usually due to a severe and prolonged deficiency of vitamin D.

Vitamin D is necessary for maintaining bone health. Adequate calcium and phosphate availability in the body is necessary for normal bone development and mineralization. Vitamin D plays an important role in promoting the absorption of calcium and phosphorus, which is necessary for bone mineralization. When calcium and phosphate levels are insufficient, vitamin D stimulates bone resorption to maintain serum calcium and phosphorus levels. However, in the case of vitamin D deficiency, there is not enough vitamin D available in the body to maintain optimum calcium and phosphorus levels, resulting in hypocalcemia and hypophosphatemia.

This deficient mineralization can lead to rickets and/or osteomalacia. Rickets occur when there is deficient mineralization in the growth plate, whereas osteomalacia is characterized by deficient mineralization of the bone matrix. These conditions cause the bones to become weak and bend over time.

Osteomalacia

Osteomalacia is a condition in adults where bones soften due to a prolonged deficiency of vitamin D. This results in impaired mineralization of bone matrix, which leads to weakened bones that are more susceptible to fractures.

Osteoporosis

Osteoporosis is a condition where the density and mass of bones decrease, or the quality and structure of bones change. This can cause bones to become weak and increase the likelihood of fractures.

Studies have found that insufficient intake of vitamin D over a prolonged period can cause demineralization of bones. A lack of vitamin D results in reduced absorption of calcium. The parathyroid glands respond by producing excess parathyroid hormone (PTH), leading to hyperparathyroidism. This eventually causes the body to extract calcium from bones to maintain calcium levels in the bloodstream. Continuous bone resorption weakens bone architecture, increasing the risk of fractures and ultimately resulting in osteoporosis and elevated fracture risk.

Cardiovascular Disease

Having low levels of vitamin D can increase your chances of developing cardiovascular diseases such as hypertension, heart failure, and ischemic heart disease. Vitamin D is important in regulating blood pressure as it hinders the secretion of renin and the activation of RAAS, which leads to a reduction in the level of angiotensin II, the main culprit in raising blood pressure. In people with vitamin D deficiency, the level of angiotensin II increases, leading to hypertension. Furthermore, heart patients suffering from severe vitamin D deficiency are at a higher risk of sudden cardiac death or heart failure compared to those with optimal levels of vitamin D.

Lower levels of vitamin D are also linked to a higher risk of diabetes. A study was conducted on individuals with impaired fasting glucose to determine the impact of vitamin D on fasting glucose levels. The study concluded that individuals with normal levels of vitamin D experienced a lesser increase in fasting glucose levels compared to those with low levels of vitamin D. This indicates that vitamin D might play a crucial role in regulating glycemic control, leading to potential benefits for cardiovascular outcomes.

Severe Asthma

Vitamin D not only can prevent asthma, but it also prevents the worsening of asthma. Low levels of Vitamin D may increase the frequency of asthma attacks and wheezing and require more medication. This is because low levels of Vitamin D can increase airway smooth muscle (ASM), causing narrowing of the airway and reducing lung function in severe asthma. To prevent and control asthma, it's important to get your daily dose of Vitamin D from natural sources like sun exposure and food. However, taking Vitamin D supplements may not produce the same results and can even worsen asthma symptoms.

Cognitive Impairment

Low Vitamin D levels can lead to a higher chance of cognitive decline. Vitamin D is a hormone that is important for the central nervous system. It helps regulate neurotransmitters and neurotrophins and has protective properties for the brain. Vitamin D also helps increase nerve growth factor levels and clears out amyloid. Studies have shown that people with cognitive impairment and dementia have lower levels of Vitamin D. It is because, when there is a deficiency of Vitamin D in the body, nerve growth factor levels decrease and amyloid accumulates, which can increase the risk of developing cognitive impairment, dementia, and Alzheimer's disease.

Cancer

Research has linked low levels of Vitamin D to various types of cancer, such as prostate, breast cancer, colon cancer, and multiple myeloma. This is because Vitamin D is known to have various biological functions that may help prevent or reduce the progression of cancer. These functions include inhibiting cancer cell growth, slowing down tumor progression, and inducing cancer cell death (apoptosis).

Autoimmune Disorders

A deficiency in Vitamin D can increase your risk of autoimmune diseases such as rheumatoid arthritis, type 1 diabetes, systemic lupus erythematosus, multiple sclerosis, and inflammatory bowel disease.

Vitamin D has the ability to regulate gene expression and inflammation, which can have a positive impact on the immune system. It has been proven to reduce the production of pro-inflammatory cytokines, enhance Treg activity, improve Natural Killer T cell function, and promote the production of anti-inflammatory cytokines. Insufficient Vitamin D intake can contribute to the development and progression of autoimmune disorders.

Infections

Research has shown that a deficiency in Vitamin D increases the risk and severity of respiratory infections such as colds, tuberculosis, pneumonia, and bronchitis. Vitamin D plays a vital role in regulating the immune system, it modulates both innate and adaptive immune responses. It also influences the production of an important antimicrobial peptide, cathelicidin.

Vitamin D helps to decrease the production of inflammation-causing cytokines while increasing the production of anti-inflammatory and anti-allergic cytokines. Furthermore, it increases the production of cathelicidin, which is an antimicrobial peptide that can directly eliminate pathogens. In addition to its role against Mycobacterium tuberculosis, cathelicidin has also been found to be effective against viruses and other bacteria.

If you are deficient in Vitamin D, your immune system becomes dysregulated and more prone to a pro-inflammatory state, which increases your susceptibility to infections caused by bacteria and viruses.

Pregnancy Complications

Maintaining normal Vitamin D levels during pregnancy is crucial for both mother's and child's health. Vitamin D aids in calcium absorption in your body, which is important for both children and adults. In the third trimester of pregnancy, there is an increase in calcium demands, making vitamin D status vital for optimal maternal health, fetal bone growth, and positive outcomes for both mother and child. If there is a deficiency of vitamin D during pregnancy, it can lead to various complications such as preeclampsia (hypertension during pregnancy), low birth weight, hypocalcemia and poor growth in the baby, weak bones, and an increased risk of autoimmune diseases.

How do I know if I am deficient in vitamin D?

It is possible to have a vitamin D deficiency without experiencing any symptoms. Here are some common symptoms associated with vitamin D deficiency:
- Fatigue and exhaustion
- Muscle cramps and muscle weakness
- Bone pain
- Mood changes, sadness, or depression
- Improper sleeping pattern
- Hair loss
- Loss of appetite

What should I do if I have symptoms of Vitamin D deficiency?

If you are experiencing exhaustion, pain in bones and muscles, or other vitamin D deficiency symptoms, consult your doctor. Your doctor might request a calcifediol blood test to check if there are any deficiencies of Vitamin D in your bloodstream.

What is a calcifediol blood test?

The blood concentration of calcifediol or 25(OH)D3 is considered the best indicator of vitamin D status, this is why the calcifediol blood test is used to determine how much actual vitamin D is in your body.

Calcifediol is measured in nanograms per milliliter (ng/mL). Different countries follow different guidelines for vitamin D intake. Some professional societies recommend a standard range of between 20 ng/mL and 40 ng/mL, while others recommend a normal range of between 30 and 50 ng/mL.

CHAPTER 4

IMPORTANCE OF VITAMIN D

FUNCTIONS OF VITAMIN D IN THE BODY

Role in Absorption of Calcium and Phosphorous

Vitamin D is crucial for strong bones. Calcium and phosphorous are essential minerals that help make bones strong. Vitamin D plays an essential role in absorbing and balancing calcium and phosphorous in the body, which enhances bone mineralization and increases bone mineral density (BMD).

Bone mineralization is the process of filling organic bones with calcium and phosphate. The higher the density of calcium and phosphate in your bones, the more robust and less prone to breaking they become.

Vitamin D primarily enhances the absorption of calcium and phosphorus in the small intestine. When calcium levels are low, Parathyroid Hormone (PTH) secretion increases, which stimulates the production of vitamin D active metabolite in the kidney. This hormone interacts with the vitamin D receptor [VDR] in the intestine, increasing calcium absorption. As a result, serum calcium and phosphorus concentrations increase, which are necessary for the mineralization of bones to prevent rickets, osteomalacia, and osteoporosis.

If normal blood calcium levels are not maintained through intestinal calcium absorption, vitamin D metabolite works with PTH to increase calcium reabsorption from the kidney and may remove calcium from the bones to maintain optimal physiological levels.

Vitamin D deficiency leads to a decrease in calcium absorption and release of calcium from the bones to maintain circulating calcium concentrations. This causes bones to weaken and become more susceptible to breaking.

Is Vitamin D an Antioxidant?

While current research studies have not confirmed vitamin D's potential role as an antioxidant, several studies have found that it effectively regulates oxidative stress. Both Vitamin D3 and Vitamin D2 can inhibit iron-dependent liposomal lipid peroxidation. Vitamin D helps to reduce oxidative stress by promoting the production of various molecules that play a role in the body's antioxidant defense system. It enhances the expression of the body's master antioxidant, Glutathione, and other antioxidant enzymes, including glutathione peroxidase and superoxide dismutase enzymes. Additionally, it suppresses the expression of free radical-producing NADPH oxidase, which helps prevent chronic diseases like diabetes, cardiovascular disease, and chronic kidney disease.

Anti-inflammatory Action

The role of Vitamin D in regulating the inflammation system is crucial. It helps control the production of inflammatory cytokines, prostaglandins, immune cells, and the nuclear factor kappa B (NF-κB) pathway, which are vital in developing immune-related diseases.

Vitamin D has powerful anti-inflammatory properties and can reduce pro-inflammatory mediators and increase anti-inflammatory cytokines. It regulates the adaptive immune system, particularly T cells, which can differentiate into pro-inflammatory TH1 cytokine cells or anti-inflammatory TH2 cytokine cells. Vitamin D suppresses inflammation causing TH1 proliferation and cytokine production while also increasing anti-inflammatory TH2 cell proliferation and cytokine production.

In addition, Vitamin D plays a crucial role in the Nuclear factor kappa B pathway (NF-κB), a major regulator of immune, stress, and inflammatory responses. The NFκB pathway can upregulate the expression of pro-inflammatory cytokines and contribute to the induction of C-reactive protein (CRP), a marker of inflammation in the body. Vitamin D can exert an anti-inflammatory effect by modulating the NFκB pathway and decreasing CRP levels. It can inhibit NF-κB activation by upregulating IκBα, the inhibitor of NF-κB, which decreases pro-inflammatory cytokine levels. Vitamin D can also inhibit the synthesis of inflammation-causing Prostaglandin E2 (PGE2).

Neuroprotective Action

Research has shown that Vitamin D plays a vital role in protecting the nervous system from injury and neurotoxicity. A deficiency in Vitamin D may increase the risk of various central nervous system (CNS) diseases such as dementia, schizophrenia, and multiple sclerosis.

Vitamin D. regulates the development and function of the nervous system It has a neuroprotective effect by influencing the production and release of growth factors neurotrophin, synthesis of neuro mediators that transmit messages between neurons, neuronal calcium regulation, an essential role in glutamatergic systems, and prevention of oxidative damage to nerve cells.

Oxidative stress is the leading cause of various neurodegenerative diseases, and Vitamin D3 has been found to alleviate oxidative stress and provide neuroprotection. It decreases lipid peroxidation, improves the GST enzyme activity, and increases the amount of reduced Glutathione, thereby reducing the effects of oxidative stress.

Immunomodulatory Effects of Vitamin D

Vitamin D has the ability to change how your immune system responds, making it an immunomodulator. Normally, the immune system fights off pathogens and foreign substances. However, sometimes, it can overreact due to a false alarm, causing an imbalance in the body and leading to autoimmune diseases. Immunomodulators help prevent this by regulating the immune system's response to achieve an immune balance.

Vitamin D's immunomodulatory effect is based on its ability to modify gene transcription. It can downregulate all adaptive immunity mechanisms, reduce inflammation, and increase immunological tolerance. Vitamin D also restricts T cell overreaction to an antigen, which impairs B cell activity and antibody production. Moreover, it influences cytokine production by reducing inflammation-causing cytokine production and stimulating immune cells to release more anti-inflammatory cytokines.

Top health benefits of getting Vitamin D from natural sources:

1. Prevent Osteoporosis

Osteoporosis is a frequently occurring bone disease among individuals who are 65 years or older. This condition arises from changes in bone mineral density and mass, which lead to a decline in bone structure and quality. This, in turn, reduces bone strength, putting individuals at a higher risk of experiencing fractures.

Osteoporosis stems from inflammation and muscle dysfunction. Elevated levels of inflammation-causing cytokines in the body are linked to increased bone metabolism. Vitamin D helps reduce the risk of bone fractures through various mechanisms, it enhances muscle strength, which helps decrease the frequency of falls, a major contributor to fractures. Additionally, vitamin D's anti-inflammatory and immunoregulatory actions help lower the production of cytokines that cause inflammation. This, in turn, reduces bone turnover and increases bone mineral density, thereby strengthening bones and minimizing fracture risk.

2. Prevent Hypertension

Vitamin D plays a vital role in regulating the renin-angiotensin-aldosterone system, thereby decreasing blood pressure by reducing the blood pressure-raising hormone, angiotensin II. Another hormone, Parathyroid hormone (PTH), increases systolic blood pressure by decreasing systemic vascular resistance, increasing heart rate, and elevating cardiac output. Vitamin D lowers PTH concentrations and leads to decreased systolic and diastolic blood pressure. However, clinical trials indicate that taking vitamin D supplements may not reduce cardiovascular risks.

3. Prevent Cardiovascular Diseases

Your vitamin D status is closely connected to your heart health and the likelihood of developing cardiovascular disease. A deficiency in vitamin D can lead to arterial stiffening, high cholesterol levels, vascular dysfunction, and an increased risk of strokes. Those with low levels of vitamin D are twice as likely to have a heart attack as those with high levels. Vitamin D helps regulate immune cells and inflammatory pathways that contribute to cardiovascular disease conditions such as atherosclerosis. Additionally, vitamin D plays a vital role in regulating cholesterol levels, one of the primary risk factors for cardiovascular disease.

Vitamin D's influence on calcium metabolism is crucial, as it promotes intestinal calcium absorption, reduces intestinal fatty acid absorption, and facilitates the conversion of cholesterol into bile acids in the liver, leading to lower cholesterol levels. Vitamin D also impacts lipoprotein metabolism, lowering triglyceride synthesis and secretion in the liver and leading to reduced triglyceride and VLDL-C levels and increased HDL-C levels (good cholesterol).

4. Lower Risk of Diabetes

Low levels of vitamin D have been linked to higher levels of inflammation in the body, which in turn could lead to insulin resistance and type 2 diabetes. Fortunately, getting enough vitamin D from natural sources can help prevent type 2 diabetes or improve insulin release and insulin sensitivity. However, clinical studies have shown that taking vitamin D supplements doesn't have a significant impact on blood sugar control. So, the diabetes-preventive benefits of vitamin D are best achieved by obtaining vitamin D from sunlight and a diet rich in vitamin D rather than from dietary supplements.

5. Prevent Cancer

Consuming high amounts of Vitamin D can significantly reduce the risk of cancer types, such as breast, prostate, and colon cancer, and lower cancer mortality rates.

Vitamin D has several biological functions that can help prevent or slow down cancer development. These include reducing cancer cell growth, decreasing tumor progression, and limiting tumor blood vessel formation (angiogenesis). Additionally, Vitamin D has anti-inflammatory and immunomodulatory effects.

When it comes to cancer-related inflammation, Vitamin D can help by decreasing levels of cyclooxygenase-2 (COX-2) enzyme, which is responsible for the production of inflammatory prostaglandins. Vitamin D also boosts the enzyme that breaks down prostaglandins, leading to decreased levels of these inflammatory mediators. Vitamin D also suppresses the activation and signaling of a protein called NFκB, which promotes inflammation and contributes to the development of cancer.

Moreover, Vitamin D can also help the immune system fight cancer by suppressing the function of Myeloid-derived suppressor cells (MDSC), which inhibit the ability of T cells to attack and remove tumor cells from the body. By reducing MDSC activity, Vitamin D can increase T-cell mediated clearance of cancer cells.

6. Prevent Rheumatoid Arthritis

The immune system's primary function is to protect the body from infections. However, in cases of autoimmune conditions such as rheumatoid arthritis, the immune system erroneously attacks the healthy cells in the joints, lungs, and other areas. Studies have shown that individuals with higher levels of vitamin D have a lower risk of developing autoimmune diseases.

This is attributed to vitamin D's ability to interact with immune cells, alter the response of the immune system, and regulate inflammation-regulating genes. Consequently, the body is better equipped to fight off sickness and disease, including arthritis.

7. Improve Eczema (Atopic Dermatitis)

Skin inflammation and immune dysfunction can lead to damage to the skin barrier and increase the likelihood of skin infections and atopic dermatitis (eczema). Vitamin D is known to have a regulatory effect on both immune function and the skin barrier.

Individuals with eczema often lack the proper production of effector cells of innate immunity, including antimicrobial peptides like cathelicidin. Vitamin D can enhance the production of cathelicidin, which boosts antimicrobial activity. Additionally, vitamin D can directly suppress skin inflammation by increasing the levels of the anti-inflammatory cytokine IL-10.

Regarding skin barrier function, vitamin D plays a regulatory role in controlling cell growth in the deepest skin layer, regulating proteins in this layer, and synthesizing lipids necessary for the skin's barrier function. Therefore, vitamin D has the potential to improve allergy outcomes through its effects on epidermal barrier function, immune regulation, and bacterial defense.

8. Promote Weight Loss:

Although there is no clear evidence that consuming higher amounts of vitamin D directly leads to weight loss, it can still help support your weight loss journey if combined with exercise and a nutritious diet. Vitamin D can affect the way fat is formed and stored in your body and increase levels of serotonin and testosterone. Serotonin is known to impact mood, emotional stability, and sleep and acts as a hunger suppressant, increasing satiety and controlling appetite. Meanwhile, testosterone plays a vital role in boosting metabolism, burning calories, and aiding in weight loss.

9. Prevent Depression and Enhance Mood

Research has shown that low vitamin D levels may be linked to anxiety and depression. This is because vitamin D is crucial in serotonin production, a neurotransmitter that elevates your mood, emotions, happiness, and sexual behavior.

10. Improve Sleep Quality

A deficiency in Vitamin D can increase your likelihood of experiencing sleep disorders. This is because Vitamin D is crucial in regulating sleep and improving the production of melatonin, which is known as the sleep hormone. Melatonin levels naturally increase in the evening, helping to calm the body and promote sleep. Ensuring that your diet includes sufficient Vitamin D-rich foods and exposure to sunlight can have a positive impact on preventing, managing, or even correcting sleep disorders. This can result in a decrease in the time it takes to fall asleep, better overall sleep quality, and longer sleep duration.

CHAPTER 5

10 NATURAL SOURCES TO GET VITAMIN D

Spending time in the early morning sunlight is the best way to your daily dose of Vitamin D. While it can be tough to get enough vitamin D from your diet alone, it's also important to eat foods high in this nutrient to avoid any deficiencies. Getting enough vitamin D is important for your health, and although sunlight exposure is the best way to achieve this, it may not always be possible to get enough during the winter months. That's why it's essential to include foods high in vitamin D in your diet. While not all foods listed below can provide enough vitamin D when taken alone, combining them can help you meet your daily requirements. Moreover, these foods offer other nutrients and fiber that can boost your overall health. Unlike supplements, there is no risk of vitamin D toxicity from either sunlight exposure or consuming foods rich in vitamin D. So, even if you're currently taking supplements for a vitamin D deficiency, it's better to switch to natural sources once your course is complete.

Below are the 10 natural sources to get vitamin D:

1. Sunlight

Many individuals aren't getting enough sunlight, perhaps due to spending more time indoors or using sunscreen when outside. However, it's important to note that sunlight is unbeatable when it comes to obtaining sufficient amounts of vitamin D. To safely receive this vitamin from the sun without risking sunburn or harmful UV radiation, follow these steps:

• It's important to get 10-25 minutes of sunlight exposure before noon, as the ultraviolet B rays with a wavelength of 290-320 nanometers during this time period are necessary for the skin to create vitamin D.

• When the skin is exposed to sunlight, it triggers the production of vitamin D within the body.

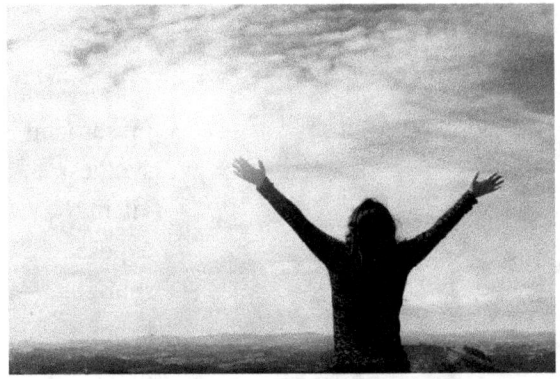

- The longer you're exposed to the sun, the more vitamin D your body produces. However, be careful not to overdo it, as excessive sunlight can lead to sunburn and other skin issues.

- It is important to have daily exposure to the sun in order to receive enough vitamin D. However if this is not possible, it is recommended to have sun exposure at least twice a week for a minimum of 25-30 minutes.

- It is recommended to get direct exposure to sunlight rather than the rays that are filtered through window glasses.

- If you want to increase your vitamin D levels while spending time in the sun, make sure to expose your face, arms, and hands or an equivalent area of your body.

- During this period, it is recommended that you avoid using sunscreen because it blocks the sun rays from entering your skin. However, remember to wear sunscreen whenever you leave home.

2. Mushrooms

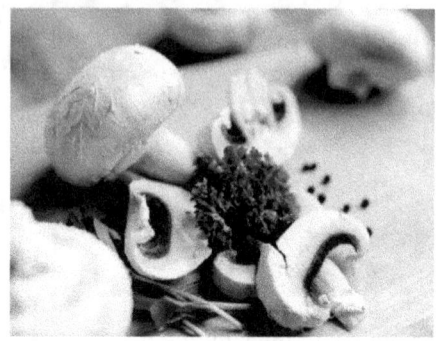

Like humans, mushrooms can synthesize vitamin D when exposed to sunlight. When exposed to UV light, the ergosterol in mushrooms is converted to vitamin D. Next time you plan to eat mushrooms, expose them to sunlight for about 10-15 minutes in the morning to make them rich in Vitamin D. You can eat fried mushrooms and can also use them as a filling for sandwiches or add to noodles.

3. Whole Cow's Milk

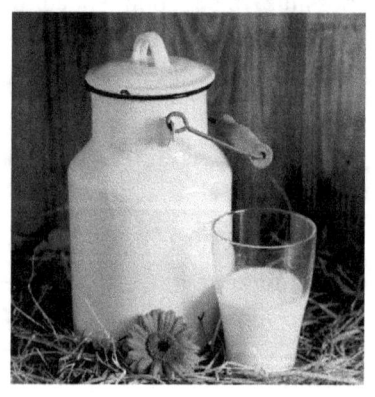

Cow's milk is considered a complete food as it contains almost all the essential nutrients. Whole milk is not only a good source of vitamin D, riboflavin, and vitamin B12, but it is also a source of complete protein and a great source of minerals such as calcium, iodine, and phosphorus.

4. Cheese

Cheese is high in calcium, protein, and fat, as well as vitamin D. It is also rich in Vitamin A, Riboflavin, and Vitamin B12. For maximum health benefits, choose the right kind of cheese.

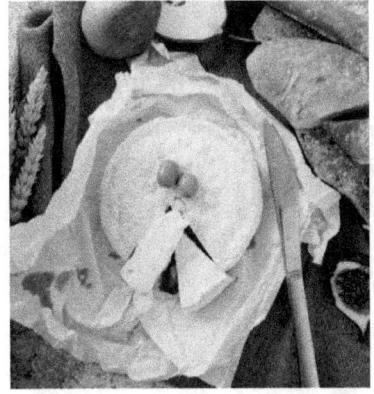

Cottage cheese, ricotta, and feta cheese are some healthier cheese options you can add to your diet. Although cheddar cheese is high in fat, it is a great source of vitamin D. 100 grams of shredded cheddar cheese contains 6% of your daily value of vitamin D.

5. Yogurt

While not the best, curd still provides a decent amount of Vitamin D. It is high in protein and lower in calories than cheese. Additionally, yogurt is a probiotic that promotes gut health. To ensure you meet your daily required vitamin D

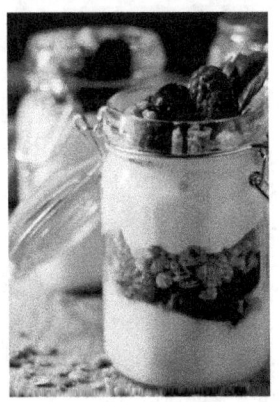

intake, consider incorporating both yogurt and milk into your diet.

6. Rice Milk

Rice milk is a great alternative to dairy milk. It is made by blending partially boiled rice, usually brown rice, with water. This milk is typically unsweetened and free of saturated fat and cholesterol. It's an ideal option for individuals with allergies who cannot consume soy or almond milk.

7. Butter

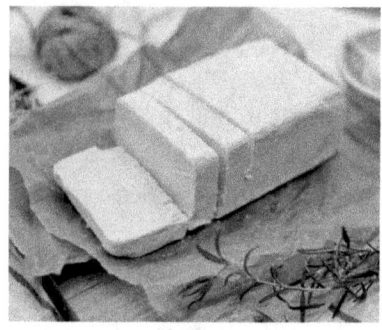

Although butter is often considered unhealthy, when consumed in moderation, it can actually be a nutritious addition to your diet. Butter contains limited vitamin D, and its saturated fat content helps the body absorb antioxidants and vitamin D from other sources. However, consuming butter in moderation is important to avoid potential health issues.

8. Milk Powder

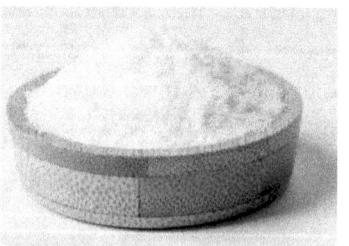

Milk powder is formed by evaporating milk until it becomes dry in order to extend its shelf life. It is packed with

Vitamin D and calcium, containing 25.6 IU per cup. Consuming milk powder in moderation is important, as excessive consumption can harm your health due to its oxidized cholesterol content, which can lead to heart-related issues.

9. Sour Cream

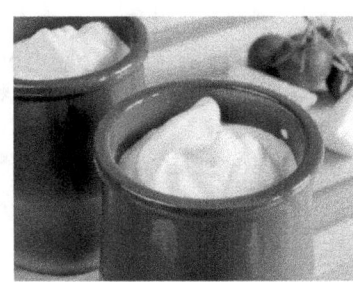

Sour cream often gets a bad reputation when it comes to health, similar to butter. However, it's important to note that sour cream is actually quite nutrient-rich. It contains essential nutrients like protein, vitamin A, potassium, and calcium and can even be a good source of vitamin D for vegetarians. Just one tablespoon of sour cream provides 2 IU of vitamin D and only 28 calories. As with any food, moderation is key, but incorporating sour cream into your diet can be a beneficial choice.

10. Other Not So Natural Sources - Fortified Foods

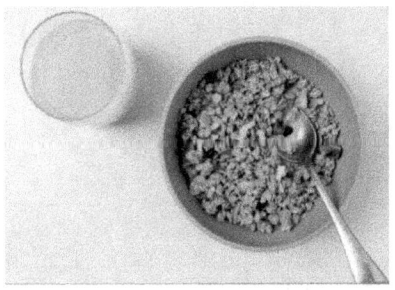

Although orange juice does not contain vitamin D, most orange juices sold in the market are fortified with it.

It is important to check the item label to determine the amount of vitamin D added.

Some cereals are fortified with vitamin D, but it may not be sufficient to meet the recommended daily intake. To fulfill your body's vitamin D needs, it is best to have cereals with cow milk. Keep in mind that fortified foods should not be your only source of vitamins, as they are not natural. While it is safe to consume them occasionally, relying solely on fortified foods to meet your body's vitamin needs is not recommended.

CHAPTER 6

POTENTIALLY DANGEROUS VITAMIN D COMBINATIONS YOU SHOULD AVOID

When taking vitamins, it's important to consider how different combinations may affect the body. For vitamins to produce their intended effects, they must be adequately absorbed in the body. Combining certain vitamins with other vitamins, medications, or minerals can either enhance or hinder their absorption rates. Some vitamin combinations may have a synergistic effect, increasing the absorption of other vitamins and providing better health benefits than if taken alone. However, other combinations may compete for absorption in the body, nullifying their effects and potentially causing toxicity.

HIGH DOSE OF VITAMIN D + MAGNESIUM

It's important to take the right amounts of Vitamin D and magnesium, even though they are an ideal combination. Taking too many Vitamin D supplements can be harmful, as it can lead to toxic levels of Vitamin D in the blood. This can result in a depletion of magnesium. However, when you get your Vitamin D from food sources or sunlight, it's less likely to reach those toxic levels. If you take high doses of Vitamin D for an extended period, it can lead to calcium build-up in the blood, which is known as hypercalcemia. This can potentially increase magnesium excretion through urine, leading to magnesium volume depletion in the body.

VITAMIN D + WATER-SOLUBLE VITAMINS

In order to receive the health benefits of vitamins, they must be properly absorbed. It's not recommended to take fat-soluble vitamins (A, D, E, and K) with water-soluble vitamins (B complex and C) because they are absorbed differently in the body. Combining them may reduce the health benefits you receive from each. Water-soluble vitamins are well absorbed on an empty stomach, while fat-soluble vitamins require the presence of fat in the body to be adequately absorbed. To maximize the benefits of each type of vitamin, consume B and C-rich foods in the morning and foods rich in A, D, E, and K in the evening. If you take vitamin supplements, take B and C on an empty stomach and take fat-soluble vitamins in the evening after a meal.

CHAPTER 7

VITAMIN D COMBINATIONS FOR SYNERGISTIC HEALTH BENEFITS

VITAMIN D + CALCIUM

You may have noticed that calcium supplements usually come in combination with vitamin D. This is because both nutrients are crucial for maintaining strong and healthy bones. Vitamin D plays a critical role in calcium absorption, increasing its absorption by two times. If your body lacks Vitamin D, it cannot efficiently absorb calcium. This results in an insufficient amount of calcium for your body's needs. Consequently, your body may extract calcium from your bones to meet its other needs, which can weaken your bones, hinder new bone growth, and increase the risk of fractures.

The relationship between vitamin D and calcium is interconnected. It's not just that vitamin D impacts the availability of calcium in the body, but calcium also affects the availability of vitamin D. Insufficient calcium intake elevates the likelihood of vitamin D deficiency. Conversely, consuming high levels of calcium guarantees that vitamin D remains available in the body for a more extended period.

To receive maximum health benefits, spend 10 to 30 minutes in the sun in the morning and follow up with a glass of milk or other calcium-rich foods like yogurt, soybeans, spinach, kale, figs, papaya, and oranges.

VITAMIN D + MAGNESIUM

Optimum intake of magnesium helps to overcome vitamin D deficiency. Studies show that increasing magnesium consumption in individuals with vitamin D deficiency can boost their vitamin D levels. Magnesium is crucial for vitamin D synthesis, activation, regulation, and transportation. Vitamin D remains inactive until it is converted by enzymes in the liver and kidney into its active form. For these enzymes to work effectively, they require magnesium. Without it, the enzymes cannot efficiently convert inactive vitamin D into its active form, and you miss out on its health benefits. In return, Vitamin D promotes magnesium absorption in the body, particularly in those with low magnesium levels.

Combining magnesium and vitamin D is crucial for optimal health as they work together to improve various functions within the body. This powerful duo strengthens the immune system, promotes healthy bone growth, and alleviates muscle spasms. Also, this life-saving combination reduces the risk of insulin resistance, type 2 diabetes, and hypertension by many folds. Magnesium-rich foods that you can combine with vitamin D are a handful of pumpkin seeds, chia seeds, cashews, peanuts, spinach, kale, brown rice, and yogurt.

VITAMIN K2 + VITAMIN D

To boost your bone health and cardiovascular health, it is recommended to consume both vitamin K and vitamin D together. These fat-soluble vitamins play an important role in calcium metabolism. When taken together, they are more effective in increasing bone density and reducing the risk of fractures compared to when taken alone. Vitamin D helps increase the concentration of bone proteins such as osteocalcin and Gla protein (BGP), which are responsible for bone formation. However, these proteins remain inactive and require vitamin K to be converted into their active form. Osteocalcin then binds to calcium and helps transport it from the blood to the bones. Without enough vitamin K and vitamin D, calcium may not be absorbed into the bone and instead get deposited in the arteries, affecting bone and cardiovascular health. Vitamin K reduces calcium excretion through urine, while vitamin D increases intestinal calcium absorption and prevents hypocalcemia. Vitamin K2 - MK-4 is effective for bone health, while MK-7 is beneficial for cardiovascular health.

Vitamin D deficiency, along with vitamin K deficiency, increases your risk of hypertension and diabetes. Having both vitamins together can help keep the blood pressure normal. Furthermore, vitamins D and K can improve insulin secretion and beta-cell proliferation in the pancreas, and provide protection against cardiovascular diseases.

For optimal results, it is advisable to obtain vitamins from diet rather than relying on dietary supplements. Overconsumption of vitamin D supplements may even increase the risk of cardiovascular diseases. This is due to the fact that excessive vitamin D intake can cause an increase in vitamin D-dependent proteins, which require vitamin K to activate. Without sufficient vitamin K, these proteins cannot be activated. Therefore, they cannot stimulate bone mineralization or inhibit soft tissue calcification. This can ultimately lead to bone fractures and cardiovascular diseases. If you are taking blood thinners like warfarin (a vitamin K antagonist) while also taking vitamin D supplements, it is crucial to consult your doctor regarding the appropriate dosage of your vitamin D supplements. To get the maximum health benefits, add more vegetables and fermented dairy into your diet for bone and cardiovascular health.

VITAMIN D + OMEGA-3 FATS

Recent research has shown that the combination of vitamin D and omega-3 fats can provide greater protection against heart attacks, strokes, and cancer, although its effectiveness for preventing these diseases in those who already have them or are at higher risk is mixed. Studies indicate that incorporating vitamin D3 and omega-3 fatty acid-rich foods into your diet, along with light exercise, can lower the risk of cancer in the general population. This combination is particularly effective for physically active individuals over the age of 70.

In addition, the combination of omega-3 fatty acids and vitamin D has a synergic impact on mental health and can enhance cognitive function by affecting the serotonin system. Serotonin is a neurotransmitter that contributes to optimism, happiness, and contentment. If your body is deficient in vitamin D and omega-3 fatty acids, it can lead to low serotonin levels, which increases the likelihood of developing psychiatric conditions such as depression, mood swings, dementia, autism, bipolar disorder, and schizophrenia. By working in conjunction with vitamin D, omega fats like docosahexaenoic acid (DHA) and eicosapentaenoic acid (EPA) help regulate serotonin levels in the brain. Vitamin D is involved in serotonin synthesis, EPA increases serotonin release, and DHA influences serotonin receptor action. Together, these factors improve serotonin levels in the body, promoting overall happiness and reducing the risk of psychiatric disorders.

Incorporate omega-3-rich foods like seaweed, flaxseed, chia seeds, walnuts, and soybean oil into your diet, and pair them with vitamin D-rich foods such as milk and milk products. Additionally, make sure to get plenty of early morning sunlight.

CHAPTER 8

DIET PLAN

Here's a 7-day diet plan to include natural sources rich in vitamins D in your diet. Repeat this diet plan every 7 days and you will never be deficient in Vitamin D.

Day 1: Sunlight exposure for 30 minutes (>100%)

Day 2: 1 cup UV-exposed cooked mushrooms with cheddar cheese + + 2 tablespoons of butter

Day 3: 1 cup fortified soy, almond, or oat milk (20%) + 2 tablespoons of butter (2%) + 15 minutes of direct sunlight exposure

Day 4: Sunlight exposure for 20 minutes + 1 cup milk with cereal (25%)

Day 5: UV exposed cooked white mushrooms 200 g (100%)

Day 6: Sunlight exposure for 10 minutes + other milk products such as yogurt, butter, cheese and milk powder

Day 7: Sunlight exposure for 20 minutes + 1 glass milk + yogurt.

CHAPTER 9

RECIPES

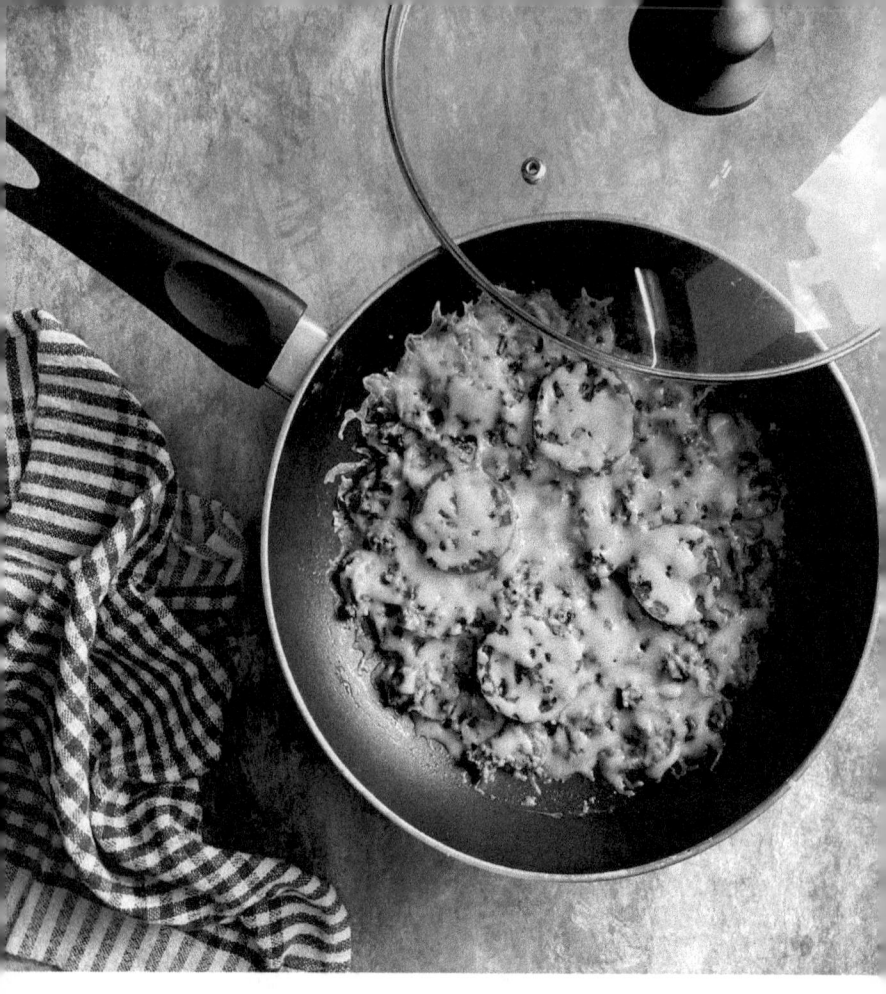

Pan Fried Cheesy Mushrooms

Ingredients

Button mushroom: 200 g   Cheddar cheese: 50 g

Cashew nuts: 30   Garlic: 5

Tomato: 1	Black pepper powder: ¼ tsp
Salt: To taste	Water: 100 ml
Butter: 1 tbsp	

Method

1. Wash and chop the mushrooms. Soak cashews in hot water for 2 hours. Grind them with water to make a thick paste.

2. Heat butter in a pan. Add chopped garlic to it and cook till it turns crisp. Take out the garlic from the pan.

3. Add chopped mushrooms, salt and black pepper powder. Cover and cook till all the water released by the mushrooms is re-absorbed.

4. Add cashew paste and mix well so that all the mushrooms get coated well in the paste. Cover with the lid and cook for 10 minutes. If it is sticking, then add 2 tbsp water.

5. Place tomato slices on top. Sprinkle salt and black pepper powder on the tomato slices. Cover and cook for 5 minutes till the tomatoes become soft.

6. Sprinkle fried garlic and shredded cheddar cheese over the mushrooms. Keep it covered for 2 minutes till the cheese melts.

7. Turn off the flame and enjoy piping hot Pan-Fried Cheesy Mushrooms.

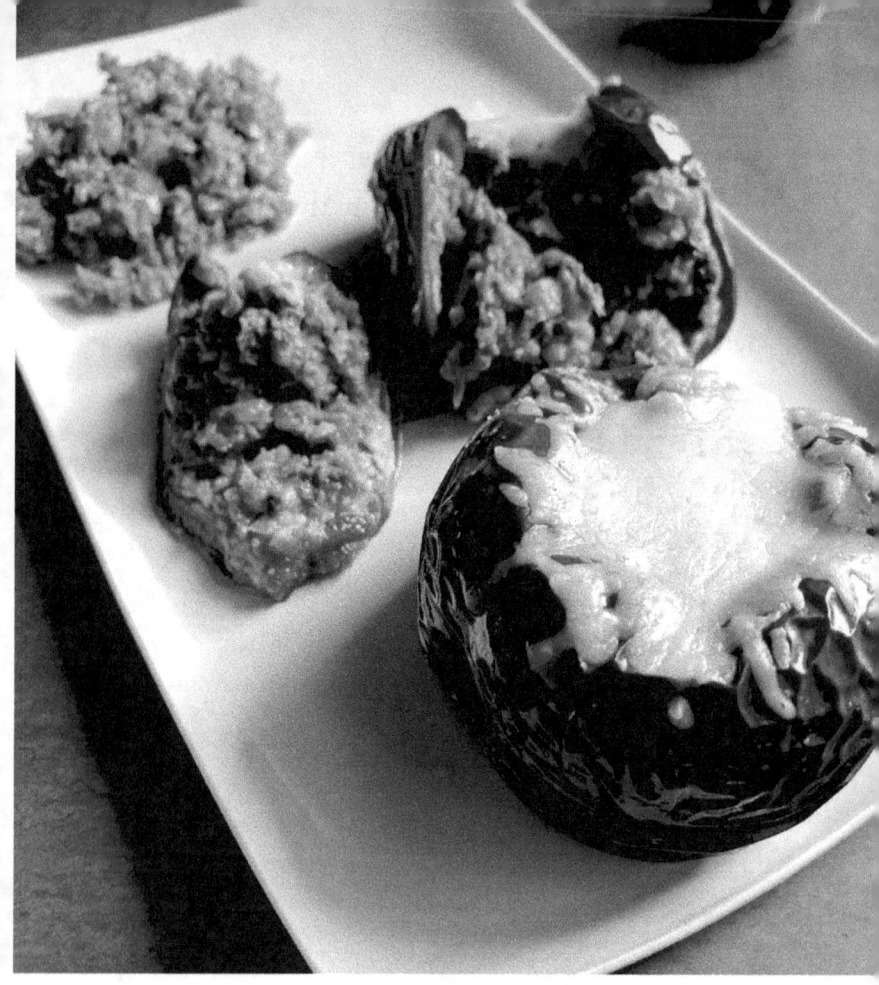

Stuffed Bell Pepper

Ingredients

Red bell pepper: 4

Cottage cheese: 200 g

Cheddar cheese: 100 g

Chopped garlic: 2 tbsp

Chopped onion: 50 g

Chopped carrot: 50 g

Chopped cabbage: 50 g	Chopped tomato: 50 g
Chopped pumpkin: 50 g	Chopped green bell
Chopped mushroom: 50 g	Mixed herbs (oregano,
Red chili pepper: ½ tsp	Salt: To taste
Oil: 2 tbsp	

Method

1. Preheat the oven to 190 °C. Heat oil in a pan. Add chopped garlic and cook for 2 minutes. Add onion and cook for 5 minutes.

2. Add all the chopped vegetables one by one and cook until mushrooms and tomato release water.

3. Add salt, red chili pepper, mixed herbs (or your choice of herbs) and mix well.

4. Lastly, add crumbled cottage cheese and cook the stuffing until it becomes slightly dry. Turn off the flame.

5. Remove the tops of the peppers and scoop out the seeds. Grease the outer side of the pepper with oil and sprinkle some salt.

6. Grate some cheese inside the pepper and fill it with the stuffing. Press the stuffing with the fingertip.

7. Place the bell peppers upside down in a baking tray and bake for 25 minutes at 190°C. Remove the peppers and sprinkle a generous amount of cheese on top. Bake again, keeping the cheese side on top for 5 minutes until the cheese is melted.

Kiwi Smoothie

Ingredients

Kiwi: 2	Papaya: 150 g / 2 slices
Curd: 100 g	Chia seeds: 1 tbsp
Ginger: ¼ inch	Black salt: To taste
Water/Coconut water: 100 ml	

Method

1. Soak chia seeds in plain water or coconut water for 2 hours.

2. Add kiwi, curd, papaya and black salt in a blender jar. Grate ginger and blend everything to make a smoothie.

3. Lastly add chia seeds and blend one last time to make a smooth kiwi smoothie.

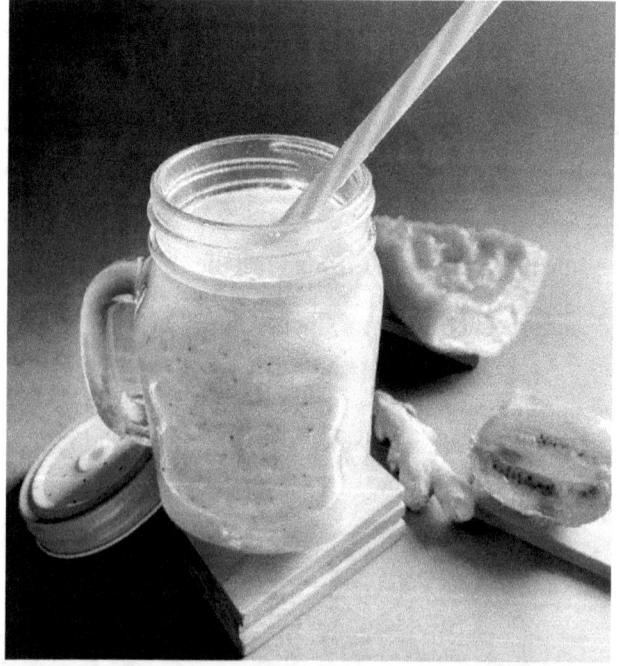

The End

Sign up to La Fonceur Newsletter to receive Bonus Recipes:

https://eatsowhat.com/signup

READ BOOKS OF THE EAT SO WHAT! SERIES

Book 1

Eat So What! Smart Ways to Stay Healthy

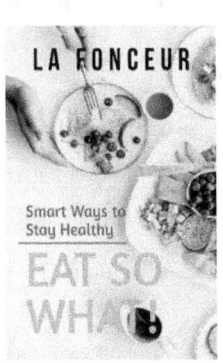

Book 2

Eat So What! The Power of Vegetarianism

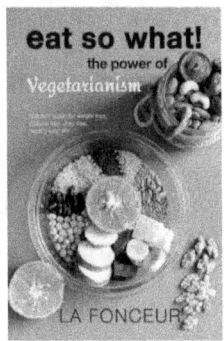

REFERENCES

1. Albahrani AA, Greaves RF. Fat-Soluble Vitamins: Clinical Indications and Current Challenges for Chromatographic Measurement. Clin Biochem Rev. 2016 Feb;37(1):27-46.

2. Multivitamin/Mineral Supplements Fact Sheet for Health Professionals, National Institutes of Health.

3. Suttie JW. Vitamin K. In: Ross AC, Caballero B, Cousins RJ, Tucker KL, Ziegler TR, eds. Modern Nutrition in Health and Disease. 11th ed. Baltimore, MD: Lippincott Williams & Wilkins; 2014:305-16.

4. Olorunnisola Olubukola Sinbad, Ajayi Ayodeji Folorunsho, Okeleji Lateef Olabisi, Oladipo Abimbola Ayoola, Emorioloye Johnson Temitope. Vitamins as Antioxidants. Journal of Food Science and Nutrition Research 2 (2019): 214-235.

5. Wiseman H. Vitamin D is a membrane antioxidant. Ability to inhibit iron-dependent lipid peroxidation in liposomes compared to cholesterol, ergosterol and tamoxifen and relevance to anticancer action. FEBS Lett 326 (1993): 285-288.

6. Food fortification overview & regional update – World Health Organisation.

7. Guidelines on food fortification with micronutrients – World Health Organisation.

8. Datta M, Vitolins MZ. Food Fortification and Supplement Use-Are There Health Implications? Crit Rev Food Sci

Nutr. 2016 Oct 2;56(13):2149-59. doi: 10.1080/10408398.2013.818527.

9. Olson R, Gavin-Smith B, Ferraboschi C, Kraemer K. Food Fortification: The Advantages, Disadvantages and Lessons from Sight and Life Programs. Nutrients. 2021 Mar 29;13(4):1118.

10. Debreceni B, Debreceni L. Role of vitamins in cardiovascular health and disease. Research Reports in Clinical Cardiology. 2014;5:283-295

11. Vitamin D Fact Sheet for Health Professionals, National Institutes of Health, Office of Dietary Supplements.

12. 25-hydroxy vitamin D test - MedlinePlus - National Library of Medicine.

13. Oliveri, Maria Beatriz, Mastaglia, Silvina Rosana; Mabel, et al.; Vitamin D3 seems more appropriate than D2 to sustain adequate levels of 25OHD: a pharmacokinetic approach; Nature Publishing Group; European Journal of Clinical Nutrition; 69; 6; 3-2015; 697-702

14. Wakeman M. A Review of the Potential Impact of Medication on Vitamin D Status. Risk Manag Health Policy. 2021 Aug 14;14:3357-3381. doi: 10.2147/RMHP.S316897.

15. Sahay M, Sahay R. Rickets-vitamin D deficiency and dependency. Indian J Endocrinol Metab. 2012 Mar;16(2):164.

16. Laird E, Ward M, McSorley E, Strain JJ, Wallace J. Vitamin D and bone health: potential mechanisms.

Nutrients. 2010 Jul;2(7):693-724. doi: 10.3390/nu2070693. Epub 2010 Jul 5.

17. Bener A, Ehlayel MS, Bener HZ, Hamid Q. The impact of Vitamin D deficiency on asthma, allergic rhinitis and wheezing in children: An emerging public health problem. J Family Community Med. 2014 Sep;21(3):154-61.

18. Jat KR, Khairwa A. Vitamin D and asthma in children: A systematic review and meta-analysis of observational studies. Lung India. 2017 Jul-Aug;34(4):355-363.

19. Sultan S, Taimuri U, Basnan SA, Ai-Orabi WK, Awadallah A, Almowald F, Hazazi A. Low Vitamin D and Its Association with Cognitive Impairment and Dementia. J Aging Res. 2020 Apr 30;2020:6097820. doi: 10.1155/2020/6097820.

20. Yang CY, Leung PS, Adamopoulos IE, Gershwin ME. The implication of vitamin D and autoimmunity: a comprehensive review. Clin Rev Allergy Immunol. 2013 Oct;45(2):217-26.

21. Gupta D, Vashi PG, Trukova K, Lis CG, Lammersfeld CA. Prevalence of serum vitamin D deficiency and insufficiency in cancer: Review of the epidemiological literature. Exp Ther Med. 2011 Mar;2(2):181-193. doi: 10.3892/etm.2011.205. Epub 2011 Jan 20.

22. Akimbekov NS, Digel I, Sherelkhan DK, Razzaque MS. Vitamin D and Phosphate Interactions in Health and Disease. Adv Exp Med Biol. 2022;1362:37-46. doi: 10.1007/978-3-030-91623-7_5. PMID: 35288871.

23. Fleet JC. The role of vitamin D in the endocrinology controlling calcium homeostasis. Mol Cell Endocrinol. 2017 Sep 15;453:36-45. doi: 10.1016/j.mce.2017.04.008. Epub 2017 Apr 9.

24. Jacquillet G, Unwin RJ. Physiological regulation of phosphate by vitamin D, parathyroid hormone (PTH) and phosphate (Pi). Pflugers Arch. 2019 Jan;471(1):83-98. doi: 10.1007/s00424-018-2231-z. Epub 2018 Nov 5.

25. Veldurthy V, Wei R, Oz L, Dhawan P, Jeon YH, Christakos S. Vitamin D, calcium homeostasis and aging. Bone Res. 2016 Oct 18;4:16041. doi: 10.1038/boneres.2016.41.

26. Laird E, Ward M, McSorley E, Strain JJ, Wallace J. Vitamin D and bone health: potential mechanisms. Nutrients. 2010 Jul;2(7):693-724. doi: 10.3390/nu2070693. Epub 2010 Jul 5.

27. Rak K, Bronkowska M. Immunomodulatory Effect of Vitamin D and Its Potential Role in the Prevention and Treatment of Type 1 Diabetes Mellitus-A Narrative Review. Molecules. 2018 Dec 24;24(1):53. doi: 10.3390/molecules24010053.

28. Chen N, Wan Z, Han SF, Li BY, Zhang ZL, Qin LQ. Effect of vitamin D supplementation on the level of circulating high-sensitivity C-reactive protein: a meta-analysis of randomized controlled trials. Nutrients. 2014 Jun 10;6(6):2206-16. doi: 10.3390/nu6062206.

29. AlJohri R, AlOkail M, Haq SH. Neuroprotective role of vitamin D in primary neuronal cortical culture.

eNeurologicalSci. 2018 Dec 17;14:43-48. doi: 10.1016/j.ensci.2018.12.004.

30. Wrzosek M, Łukaszkiewicz J, Wrzosek M, Jakubczyk A, Matsumoto H, Piątkiewicz P, Radziwoń-Zaleska M, Wojnar M, Nowicka G. Vitamin D and the central nervous system. Pharmacol Rep. 2013;65(2):271-8.

31. Prisant LM, Gujral JS, Mulloy AL. Hyperthyroidism: a secondary cause of isolated systolic hypertension. J Clin Hypertens (Greenwich). 2006 Aug;8(8):596-9.

32. Fisher SB, Perrier ND. Primary hyperparathyroidism and hypertension. Gland Surg. 2020 Feb;9(1):142-149.

33. Lips P, Eekhoff M, van Schoor N, Oosterwerff M, de Jongh R, Krul-Poel Y, Simsek S. Vitamin D and type 2 diabetes. J Steroid Biochem Mol Biol. 2017 Oct;173:280-285.

34. Palmer D. Vitamin D and the Development of Atopic Eczema. J Clin Med. 2015 May 20;4(5):1036-548.

35. Abboud M. Vitamin D Supplementation and Sleep: A Systematic Review and Meta-Analysis of Intervention Studies. Nutrients. 2022 Mar 3;14(5):1076. doi: 10.3390/nu14051076.

36. Laird E, Ward M, McSorley E, Strain JJ, Wallace J. Vitamin D and bone health: potential mechanisms. Nutrients. 2010 Jul;2(7):693-724. doi: 10.3390/nu2070693. Epub 2010 Jul 5.

37. Krishnan AV, Trump DL, Johnson CS, Feldman D. The role of vitamin D in cancer prevention and treatment.

Endocrinol Metab Clin North Am. 2010 Jun;39(2):401-18, table of contents.

38. Vitamin D and Cancer, National Cancer Institute.

39. Garland CF, Garland FC, Gorham ED, Lipkin M, Newmark H, Mohr SB, Holick MF. The role of vitamin D in cancer prevention. Am J Public Health. 2006 Feb;96(2):252-61.

40. Uchiyama K, Kishi H, Komatsu W, Nagao M, Ohhira S, Kobashi G. Lipid and Bile Acid Dysmetabolism in Crohn's Disease. J Immunol Res. 2018 Oct 1;2018:7270486.

41. Rosca MG, Vazquez EJ, Kern TS, Hoppel CL. Oxidation of fatty acids is source of increased mitochondrial reactive oxygen species production in kidney cortical tubules in early diabetes. Diabetes. 2012 Aug;61(8):2074-83. Epub 2012 May 14.

42. Koh ES, Kim SJ, Yoon HE, Chung JH, Chung S, Park CW, Chang YS, Shin SJ. Association of blood manganese level with diabetes and renal dysfunction: a cross-sectional study of the Korean general population. BMC Endocr Disord. 2014 Mar 8;14:24. doi: 10.1186/1472-6823-14-24.

43. Jandacek RJ. Linoleic Acid: A Nutritional Quandary. Healthcare (Basel). 2017 May 20;5(2):25. doi: 10.3390/healthcare5020025.

44. Wang T, Liu YY, Wang X, Yang N, Zhu HB, Zuo PP. Protective effects of octacosanol on 6-hydroxydopamine-induced Parkinsonism in rats via regulation of ProNGF

and NGF signaling. Acta Pharmacol Sin. 2010 Jul;31(7):765-74.

45. Cologne, Germany: Institute for Quality and Efficiency in Health Care (IQWiG); 2006-. What are blood thinners (anti-clotting medication) and how are they used? 2013 Nov 25 [Updated 2017 Oct 5].

46. Gary K. Schwartz, Manish A. Shah. Targeting the Cell Cycle: A New Approach to Cancer Therapy. Journal of Clinical Oncology 2005. PG 9408-9421.

47. Office of the Surgeon General (US). Bone Health and Osteoporosis: A Report of the Surgeon General. Rockville (MD): Office of the Surgeon General (US); 2004. 2, The Basics of Bone in Health and Disease.

48. CFR - Code of Federal Regulations Title 21 - US Food & Drug Administration.

49. Khatun H, Rahman A, Biswas M, Islam AU. Water-soluble Fraction of Abelmoschus esculentus L Interacts with Glucose and Metformin Hydrochloride and Alters Their Absorption Kinetics. ISRN Pharm. 2011;2011:260537. doi: 10.5402/2011/260537. Epub 2011 Sep 11.

50. Fan Y, Adam TJ, McEwan R, Pakhomov SV, Melton GB, Zhang R. Detecting Signals of Interactions Between Warfarin and Dietary Supplements in Electronic Health Records. Stud Health Technol Inform. 2017;245:370-374.

51. Reddy P, Edwards LR. Magnesium Supplementation in Vitamin D Deficiency. Am J Ther. 2019

Jan/Feb;26(1):e124-e132. doi: 10.1097/MJT.0000000000000538.

52. Toribio RE, Kohn CW, Rourke KM, Levine AL, Rosol TJ. Effects of hypercalcemia on serum concentrations of magnesium, potassium, and phosphate and urinary excretion of electrolytes in horses. Am J Vet Res. 2007 May;68(5):543-54. doi: 10.2460/ajvr.68.5.543

53. Uwitonze AM, Razzaque MS. Role of Magnesium in Vitamin D Activation and Function. J Am Osteopath Assoc. 2018 Mar 1;118(3):181-189. doi: 10.7556/jaoa.2018.037.

54. Deng X, Song Y, Manson JE, et al. Magnesium, vitamin D status and mortality: results from US National Health and Nutrition Examination Survey (NHANES) 2001 to 2006 and NHANES III. BMC Med. 2013 Aug 27;11:187.

55. Al Alawi AM, Majoni SW, Falhammar H. Magnesium and Human Health: Perspectives and Research Directions. Int J Endocrinol. 2018;2018:9041694.

56. Lips P. Interaction between vitamin D and calcium. Scand J Clin Lab Invest Suppl. 2012;243:60-4. doi: 10.3109/00365513.2012.681960.

57. Khazai N, Judd SE, Tangpricha V. Calcium and vitamin D: skeletal and extraskeletal health. Curr Rheumatol Rep. 2008 Apr;10(2):110-7. doi: 10.1007/s11926-008-0020-y.

58. Lu, T.; Shen, Y.; Wang, J.H.; Xie, H.K.; Wang, Y.F.; Zhao, Q.; Zhou, D.-Y.; Shahidi, F. Improving oxidative stability of flaxseed oil with a mixture of antioxidants. J. Food Proc. Preserv. 2020, 44, e14355.

References

59. Floros S, Toskas A, Vareltzis P. Bioaccessibility, Oxidative Stability of Omega-3 Fatty Acids in Supplements, Sardines and Enriched Eggs Studied Using a Static In Vitro Gastrointestinal Model. Molecules. 2022 Jan 9;27(2):415. doi: 10.3390/molecules27020415.

60. Bischoff-Ferrari HA, Willett WC, Manson JE, Gaengler S. Combined Vitamin D, Omega-3 Fatty Acids, a Simple Home Exercise Program May Reduce Cancer Risk Among Active Adults Aged 70 and Older: A Randomized Clinical Trial. Front Aging. 2022 Apr 25;3:852643. doi: 10.3389/fragi.2022.852643.

61. Omega 3 fatty acids fact sheet – Health Professional Fact Sheet. National Institutes of Health Office of Dietary Supplements.

62. Patrick RP, Ames BN. Vitamin D and the omega-3 fatty acids control serotonin synthesis and action, part 2: relevance for ADHD, bipolar disorder, schizophrenia, and impulsive behavior. FASEB J. 2015 Jun;29(6):2207-22. doi:10.1096/fj.14-268342.

ABOUT THE AUTHOR

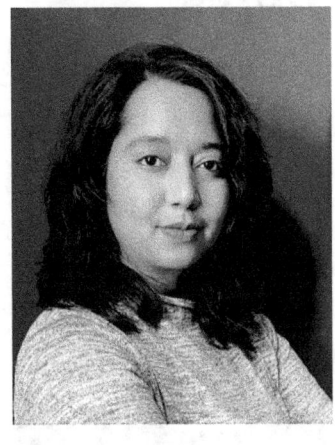

With a Master's Degree in Pharmacy, the author La Fonceur is a Research Scientist and Registered Pharmacist. She specialized in Pharmaceutical Technology and worked as a research scientist in the pharmaceutical research and development department. She is a health blogger and a dance artist. Her previous books include Eat to Prevent and Control Disease, Secret of Healthy Hair, and Eat So What! series. Being a research scientist, she has worked closely with drugs and based on her experience, she believes that one can prevent most of the diseases with nutritious vegetarian foods and a healthy lifestyle.

READ MORE FROM LA FONCEUR

English Editions | Hindi Editions

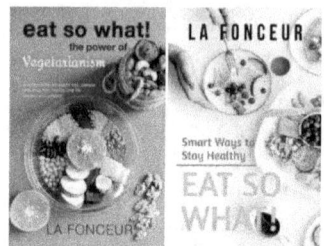
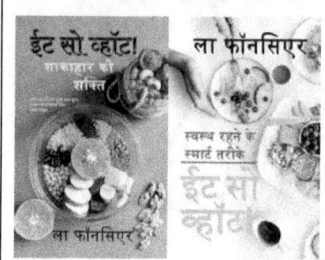

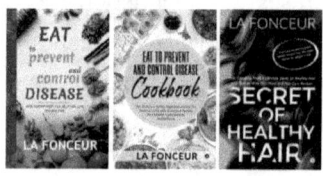
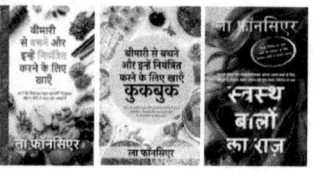

CONNECT WITH LA FONCEUR

Instagram: @la_fonceur | @eatsowhat

Facebook: LaFonceur | eatsowhatblog

Twitter: @la_fonceur

Follow on Bookbub: @eatsowhat

Sign up to get exclusive offers on La Fonceur books:

Blog: http://www.eatsowhat.com/

Website: http://www.lafonceurbooks.com/

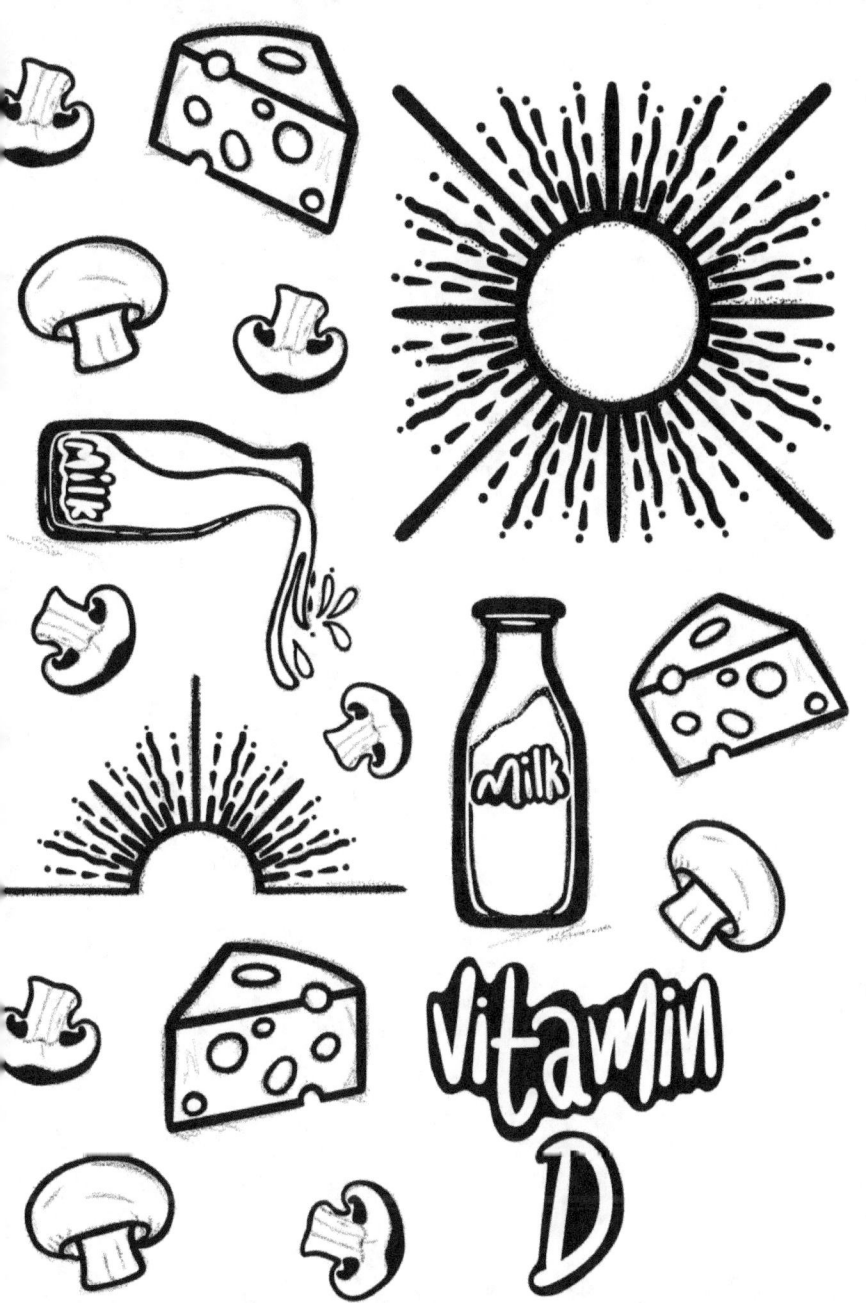

COLOR YOUR VITAMIN D

www.ingramcontent.com/pod-product-compliance
Lightning Source LLC
LaVergne TN
LVHW010428070526
838199LV00066B/5966